D-Crush Formula

Tested natural and efficient ways to lose weight faster.

By Dr. Elixir Kings

Dedicated to my family and friends as well
my great country, USA.

Table of contents

Chapter 1

Barely any years back, I used to be so fat. My companions chuckled at me due to my body size. I was generally called "Jam pot", so I had to take critical steps to look better. I realize it will work for every individual who needs a fit body like a competitor. Look hot you know.. so how about we hit it.

Food Equation

1. Add Protein to Your Eating regimen Oftentimes

With regards to weight reduction, protein is the ruler of supplements.

Your body consumes calories while processing and utilizing the protein you eat, so a high-protein diet can help digestion by up to 80-100 calories each day.

A high-protein diet can likewise cause you to feel all the more full and diminish your hunger. As a matter of fact, a few investigations show that individuals eat north of 400 less calories each day on a high-protein diet.

Indeed, even something as straightforward as having a high-protein breakfast (like eggs) can make a strong difference.

2. Eat Entire, Single-Fixing Food sources

Quite possibly everything you can manage to become better is to put together your eating regimen with respect to entire, single-fixing food sources.

By doing this, you dispose of by far most of added sugar, added fat and handled food.

Most entire food sources are normally very filling, making it significantly more straightforward to keep inside solid calorie limits.

Moreover, eating entire food varieties additionally gives your body the numerous fundamental supplements that it needs to appropriately work.

Weight reduction frequently follows as a characteristic symptom of eating entire food sources.

3. Keep away from Handled Food varieties Handled food sources are generally high in added sugars, added fats and calories.

Likewise, handled food varieties are designed to cause you to eat however much as could be expected. They are significantly more prone to cause habit-forming like eating than natural food sources.

4. Stock Up on Quality Food sources and Tidbits

Studies have shown that the food you keep at home significantly influences weight and eating conduct.

By continuously having good food accessible, you decrease the possibilities of you or other relatives eating undesirable food.

There are additionally numerous solid and normal tidbits that are not difficult to plan and take with you in a hurry.

These incorporate yogurt, entire organic products, nuts, carrots,and hard-bubbled eggs.

5. Limit Your Admission of Added Sugar

Eating a ton of added sugar is connected with a portion of the world's driving illnesses, including coronary illness, type 2 diabetes and disease.

All things considered, Americans eat around 15 teaspoons of added sugar every day. This sum is typically concealed in different handled food varieties, so you might be eating a ton of sugar without acknowledging it.

Since sugar goes by many names in fixing records, sorting out how much sugar an item really contains can be extremely challenging.

Limiting your admission of added sugar is an incredible method for working on your eating routine.

6. Hydrate
There is really truth to the case that drinking water can assist with weight reduction.

Drinking 0.5 liters (17 oz) of water might expand the calories you consume by 24-30% for an hour a short time later.

Drinking water before feasts may likewise prompt diminished calorie consumption, particularly for moderately aged and more established individuals.

Water is especially great for weight reduction when it replaces different drinks that are high in calories and sugar.

7. Drink (Unsweetened) Espresso
Luckily, individuals are understanding that espresso is a sound drink that is stacked with cell reinforcements and other gainful mixtures.

Espresso drinking might uphold weight reduction by expanding energy levels and how much calories you consume.

Stimulated espresso might support your digestion by 3-11% and diminish your gamble of creating type 2 diabetes by an incredible 23-half.

Besides, dark espresso is very weight reduction cordial, since it can encourage you yet contains practically no calories.

8. Supplement With Glucomannan
Glucomannan is one of a few weight reduction pills that has been demonstrated to work.

This water-solvent, regular dietary fiber comes from the foundations of the konjac plant, otherwise called the elephant sweet potato.

Glucomannan is low in calories, occupies room in the stomach and postpones stomach exhaustion. It additionally lessens the assimilation of protein and fat, and feeds the helpful stomach microbes.

Its excellent capacity to assimilate water is accepted to be what makes it so powerful for weight reduction. One case can transform a whole glass of water into gel.

9. Stay away from Fluid Calories
Fluid calories come from refreshments like sweet sodas, organic product juices, chocolate milk and caffeinated drinks.

These beverages are awful for wellbeing in more than one way, including an expanded gamble of heftiness. One review showed an uncommon 60% expansion in the gamble of weight among youngsters, for every day to day serving of a sugar-improved drink.
It's likewise essential to take note of that your mind doesn't enlist fluid calories the same way it does strong calories, so you wind up including these calories on top of all the other things that you eat.

10. Limit Your Admission of Refined Carbs

Refined carbs will be carbs that have had the vast majority of their useful supplements and fiber eliminated.

The refining system leaves only effectively processed carbs, which can expand the gamble of indulging and infection.

The super dietary wellsprings of refined carbs are white flour, white bread, white rice, soft drinks, cakes, snacks, desserts, pasta, breakfast cereals, and added sugar.

11. Quick Irregularly
Irregular fasting is an eating design that cycles between times of fasting and eating.

There are a couple ways of doing irregular fasting, including the 5:2 eating routine, the 16:8 technique and the eat-stop-eat strategy.

By and large, these strategies cause you to eat less calories generally, without having to intentionally limit calories during the eating time frames. This ought to prompt weight reduction, as well as various other medical advantages.

12. Drink (Unsweetened) Green Tea
Green tea is a characteristic drink that is stacked with cell reinforcements.

Drinking green tea is connected with many advantages, like expanded fat consumption and weight reduction.

Green tea might increment energy use by 4% and increment particular fat consumption by to 17%, particularly harmful gut fat.

Matcha green tea is an assortment of powdered green tea that might have considerably more impressive medical advantages than normal green tea.

Search for green tea and matcha green tea on the web.

13. Eat More Products of the soil
Products of the soil are very sound, weight reduction cordial food varieties.

As well as being high in water, supplements and fiber, they generally have exceptionally low energy thickness. This makes it conceivable to eat huge servings without consuming an excessive number of calories.

Various investigations have shown that individuals who eat more leafy foods will generally weigh less.

14. Include Calories Sometimes
Monitoring what you're eating is exceptionally useful while attempting to get more fit.

There are a few powerful methods for doing this, including counting calories, keeping a food journal or taking pictures of what you eat.

Utilizing an application or another electronic device might be significantly more useful than writing in a food journal.

15. Utilize More modest Plates
A few examinations have shown that utilizing more modest plates assists you with eating less, in light of the fact that it changes how you see segment sizes.

Individuals appear to fill their plates with something very similar, paying little mind to plate size, so they wind up putting more food on bigger plates than more modest ones.

Utilizing more modest plates diminishes how much food you eat, while providing you with the view of having eaten more.

16. Attempt a Low-Carb Diet

Many investigations have shown that low-carb abstains from food are extremely viable for weight reduction.

sleepricting carbs and eating more fat and protein lessens your hunger and assists you with eating less calories.

This can bring about weight reduction that really depends on multiple times more prominent than that from a standard low-fat eating regimen.

A low-carb diet can likewise further develop many gambling factors for illness.

17. Eat All the more Leisurely
Assuming you eat excessively quickly, you might eat such a large number of calories before your body even understands that you are full.

Quicker eaters are substantially more liable to foster weight, contrasted with the individuals who eat all the more leisurely.

Biting all the more leisurely may assist you with eating less calories and increment the creation of chemicals that are connected to weight reduction.

18. Add Eggs to Your Eating regimen
Eggs are a definitive weight reduction food. They are modest, low in calories, high in protein and stacked with a wide range of supplements.

High-protein food varieties have been displayed to diminish craving and increment completion, contrasted with food varieties that contain less protein.

Besides, having eggs for breakfast might cause up to 65% more noteworthy weight reduction north of about two months, contrasted with having bagels for breakfast.

It might likewise assist you with eating less calories all through the remainder of the day.

19. Enliven Your Feasts
Stew peppers and jalapenos contain a compound called capsaicin, which might support digestion and increase the consumption of fat.

Capsaicin may likewise decrease craving and calorie consumption.

20. Take Probiotics
Probiotics are live microbes that have medical advantages when eaten. They can work on stomach related wellbeing and heart wellbeing, and may try and assist with weight reduction.

Studies have shown that individuals who are overweight and individuals who have stoutness will quite often have different stomach microorganisms than ordinary

weight individuals, which might impact weight.
Probiotics might assist with controlling the sound stomach microbes. They may likewise hinder the ingestion of dietary fat, while diminishing craving and irritation.

21. Get Sufficient sleep
Getting sufficient sleep is amazingly significant for weight reduction, as well as to fosleepall future weight gain.

Studies have shown that sleepless individuals ultimately depend on 55% bound to
foster heftiness, contrasted with the individuals who get sufficient sleep. This number is considerably higher for youngsters.

This is somewhat in light of the fact that lack of sleep upsets the day to day changes in hunger chemicals, prompting an unfortunate craving guideline.

22. Eat More Fiber
Fiber-rich food sources might assist with
weight reduction.

Food sources that contain water-solvent
fiber might be particularly useful, since this
kind of fiber can assist with expanding the
sensation of totality.

Fiber might defer stomach purging, cause
the stomach to extend and advance the
arrival of satiety chemicals.

Eventually, this causes us to eat less
normally, without mulling over everything.

Moreover, many sorts of fiber can take care
of the amicable stomach microbes. Solid
stomach microscopic organisms have been
connected with a diminished gamble of
corpulence.

Simply make a point to build your fiber consumption step by step to keep away from stomach inconvenience, for example, swelling, spasms and the runs.

23. Clean Your Teeth After Dinners
Many individuals clean or floss their teeth in the wake of eating, which might assist with sleepricting the craving to nibble or eat between dinners.

This is on the grounds that many individuals don't want to eat after cleaning their teeth. In addition, it can make food taste awful.

Accordingly, on the off chance that you brush or use mouthwash in the wake of eating, you might be less enticed to snatch a superfluous tidbit.

24. Battle Your Food Dependence
Food dependence includes overwhelming desires and changes in your mind science

that make it harder to oppose eating specific food sources.

This is a significant reason for gorging for some individuals, and influences a huge level of the populace. Truth be told, a new 2014 investigation discovered that practically 20% of individuals satisfied the standards for food habits.

A few food sources are significantly more prone to cause side effects of compulsion than others. This incorporates exceptionally handled low quality foods that are high in sugar, fat or both.

The most ideal way to beat food habits is to look for help.

25. Hit the treadmill
Hitting the treadmill — whether it is running, running, cycling, power strolling or climbing — is an incredible method for

consuming calories and working on both mental and actual wellbeing.

Cardio has been displayed to further develop many gambling factors for coronary illness. It can likewise assist with diminishing body weight.

Cardio is by all accounts especially powerful at lessening the risky gut fat that develops around your organs and causes metabolic illness.

26. Add Obstruction Activities
Loss of bulk is a typical result of eating fewer carbs.

On the off chance that you lose a great deal of muscle, your body will begin consuming less calories than previously.

By lifting loads routinely, you'll have the option to fosleepall this misfortune in bulk.

As an additional advantage, you'll likewise look and feel far improved.

27. Use Whey Protein
A great many people get sufficient protein from diet alone. Be that as it may, for the people who don't, taking a whey protein supplement is a successful method for helping protein consumption.

One review demonstrates the way that supplanting part of your calories with whey protein can cause huge weight reduction, while likewise expanding slender bulk.

Simply make a point to peruse the fixings list, since certain assortments are stacked with added sugar and other unfortunate added substances.

28. Practice Careful Eating
Careful eating is a strategy used to increment mindfulness while eating.

It assists you with pursuing cognizant food decisions and fostering attention to your craving and satiety prompts. It then assists you with eating solid in light of those prompts.

Careful eating has been displayed to altogether affect weight, eating conduct and stress in people with heftiness. It is particularly useful against pigging out and profound eating. By settling on cognizant food decisions, expanding your mindfulness and paying attention to your body, weight reduction ought to follow normally and without any problem.

29. Center around Changing Your Way of life
Eating less junk food is something that quite often flops in the long haul. As a matter of fact, individuals who "diet" will generally put on more weight after some time.

Rather than zeroing in just on shedding pounds, make it an essential objective to sustain your body with good food and supplements.

Eat to turn into a better, more joyful, fitter individual — not simply to shed pounds.

Chapter 2

Workout formula

1. Working out with Rope
The consume: 667-990 calories/hour
(bouncing at 120 skips each moment)

That's right, this impact from your jungle gym past is a complete torcher. Besides, "working out with rope is perfect for creating coordination, calf and lower leg strength, center strength, act, and cardiovascular perseverance," says Gabbi Berkow, CPT, a fitness coach and nutritionist. "It likewise assists work with boning thickness, which prepares for bone misfortune, osteoporosis, and bone misfortune."

Preferably, the most effective way to begin working out with rope is to go sluggish and do it in 20-to 30-second explodes. Whenever you've dominated that flick-of-the-wrist and your timing, work on speeding up and length to consume more calories.

For a full-body exercise challenge, give this calorie-burning leap rope exercise an opportunity.

2. Hikers
It is a focused energy practice that helps consume a ton of calories yet additionally assuming that done right further develops center strength and soundness. This is one action that can be added to any exercise

routine daily practice. 3 sets, 40 seconds on
and 20 seconds off.

Get into a board position.
Hands shoulder width separated, back
straight center locked in.
Carry your right knee to your chest to the
furthest extent that you would be able.
Switch legs and rehash the development.

3. Bodyweight invert jumps

Works on hip soundness and leg strength.
Can be added to an exercise in this style - 4
sets, 10 reps.

Begin with feet shoulder width separated.
Keeping your center tight and thrust down
with keeping one leg behind the other.
From here use leg drive to come to the
standing position. Rehash a similar on the
opposite side too.
Rehash this cycle for the endorsed reps.

4. Spreads
Chips away at further developing center, shoulder, and leg drive. Can be added to the exercise in this style - 5 sets, 7 reps, 20 seconds off
Here is a definite bit by bit clarification of spreads:

Stand up standing with knees marginally twisted.
Twist down quickly into a board position, from here kick and bring the feet near your hands.
From this position, kick back and take the feet back to board position. Rehash this for the recommended time. Get back to the beginning position.

Chapter 3

Power of Sleep

Indeed, even the best eating routine and long stretches of activity won't assist you with shedding pounds on the off chance that you don't get 7 to 8 hours of continuous sleep.

Lack of sleep influences significant chemicals that are fundamental to shed pounds. Low number of dozing hours diminishes leptin (satiety chemical), increases ghrelin (hunger chemical), and furthermore shoots up cortisol (the pressure chemical). Without enough sleep, these chemicals will leave whack, you would awaken with an inability to burn calories and an eager hunger, causing you to long for sweet and fatty food varieties on the grounds that your cerebrum is searching for moment energy to compensate for the absence of sleep. Likewise, absence of sleep makes such food more pleasurable. Rattling off them each of the individually:

1. Insulin Obstruction: Insulin, which is a glucose controlling chemical, likewise assumes a functioning part in guiding calories to be put away as glycogen and fat in muscles and tissues. At the point when there is a high measure of glucose flowing in the circulation system consistently, after a point, body cells become less receptive to the endeavors of insulin.

At the point when that occurs, all extra circling glucose is coordinated to be put away as muscle to fat ratio. Constant sleeplessness expands the gamble of insulin obstruction and dials back the rate at which one consumes calories.

2. Builds Prize Looking for Conduct: As referenced above, absence of sleep illuminates your mind's award community in light of food - in straightforward words - you would need to marshal an immense measure of resolution to say "no" to that second cut of pizza!

3. Expands Pressure Chemical Cortisol: Presently, here's the one-two punch - lack of sleep likewise builds the degree of stress chemical "cortisol," which causes weight gain, slows down weight reduction, and increments gut fat.

4. Hard To Practice Discretion: Moreover, absence of sleep dulls out action of the cerebrum, which is answerable for navigation and drive control, and that implies despite the fact that you realize that debauched piece of red velvet cake is high in calories and not great for weight reduction, you actually would feel free to have it!

5. Expands Chances of Evening Nibbling: Since you are remaining conscious for the significant piece of night, your desires for evening time eating, low quality food, and stuff high in calories, refined carbs, unfortunate fat increments.

6. Plunge in Digestion: The principal explanation for a languid digestion - absence of sleep! Hence, sleep is certainly fundamental for a sound living, particularly, for weight reduction.

7. Plunge in Fat Oxidation: Lacking sleep can plunge down fat oxidation and fat digestion - and that implies less possibilities of fat getting changed over into energy, and harder for the body to dissolve away excess fat.

9. Diminishes Muscle Union: Those of you longing for developing muscles and biceps - there's a most recent review that demonstrates the way that lack of sleep can decrease muscle protein combination by 18%!

10. Excessively Depleted For Exercise the Following Day: This is an undeniable result - since you would awaken low on energy the

following day, assembling the inspiration to exercise and exercise would be truly hard.

11. Expands Desires for High-Carb Food sources: Low number of dozing hours upgrades the gluttonous improvement handling in the cerebrum prompting expanded food consumption.

To Get a decent night's sleep - avoid blue light one hour before sleep since openness to light and blue light from contraptions can upset the circadian mood of the body. Likewise, make it a highlight to eat no less than a few hours before sleep in light of the fact that having dinnertime and sleep time excessively near one another keeps the stomach related framework dynamic and keeps you from having a decent night's sleep. Additionally, calories from the food wouldn't get used at all on the grounds that the digestion is low, and a large portion of it would get put away as fat in the body. Likewise, have some espresso or green tea a couple of hours prior to raising a ruckus around town.

With these framed strategies I want to believe that you can accomplish your weight reduction and trim down to your ideal size.

Do well to impart to loved ones. Much obliged to you.